TEST YOUR KNOWLEDGE
MCQs
THE PATIENT WITH A LOCOMOTOR DISORDER

Anne Betts, BSc(Hons),
Course Tutor,
Institute of Advanced Nursi
Royal College of N

GW00729103

Cynthia Gilling, SRN, SCM, RNT
Director of Nurse Education,
The Royal Free Hospital,
London

Marjorie Read, BA, SRN, RNT, Dip.N.
Assistant Director of Nurse Education,
The Princess Alexandra School of Nursing,
The London Hospital,
London

Maureen Theobald, MA, SRN, RCNT, RNT, Dip.Ed.
Assistant Director of Nurse Education,
The Princess Alexandra School of Nursing,
The London Hospital,
London

Harper & Row, Publishers
London

Cambridge
Hagerstown
Philadelphia
New York

San Francisco
Mexico City
São Paulo
Sydney

Harper & Row Ltd
28 Tavistock Street
London WC2E 7PN

British Library Cataloguing in Publication Data

The Patient with a locomotor disorder.—(test your knowledge)
  1. Movement disorders
  I. Betts, Anne   II. Series
  616.7'0024613   RC925.5

  ISBN 0—06—318225—6

Typeset by Gedset Limited, Cheltenham.
Printed and bound by A Wheaton & Co, Exeter.

For Pat Barry, our invaluable
secretary who still talks to us!

CONTENTS

PREFACE

This is the fifth book in the series and the last one for us as a group. Some of us have moved away to other posts and others have different commitments and it becomes increasingly more difficult to meet and produce the material required. We are very pleased that four colleagues from The Princess Alexandra School of Nursing have come forward to write the final books in the series and we wish them as much enjoyment in their writing as we have had.

The aim of the series will continue in promoting the principle of 'stories' related to patients with similar conditions but with widely differing needs.

At this time, when we have heard that the Statutory Body intends to work towards the implementation of a new examination system, we could be feeling that the 'era' of multiple choice questions is passing. Far from it, we believe it is one of the valid methods of testing knowledge and, because of its now well established use, we can see it continuing as a valuable revision tool for the foreseeable future, promoting learning and testing understanding.

The concept that questions provoke answers but multiple choice questions stimulate discussion, in order to arrive at the correct answer thus enhancing the problem-solving approach to patient-centred nursing, is firmly established. It is the primary skill involved in giving individualized patient care. This approach is the foundation of present day nursing in this country and will be the basis on which nursing competence is assessed in the future.

We are grateful to all the students and their tutors in several schools of nursing who have helped us by working through the questions for us and aiding us in the validation process. They were appreciative of the opportunity to practise and we hope you will be too. We thank all those who have made constructive comments on our work and hope that by now they will have been suitably encouraged to write and validate their own questions.

How to use this book

Each question starts with a brief 'story' about the patient, followed by a series of related multiple choice questions.

It will be necessary to refer back to the story when selecting your answer, bearing in mind the individuality of the patient and the need to assess the effect that this may have on the care planned.

It is our belief that there is only one right answer to each question, and we have given our reasons for selecting this as the most appropriate answer in a section at the end of the book.

EXAMPLE

Richard Franks is a 49-year-old bachelor who has suffered from rheumatoid arthritis for 9 years. He has been admitted to your ward during an acute phase of his disease and appears in pain and rather depressed.

1 Which one of the following should be prescribed for Mr Franks?
Bed rest:
(a) for the first 48 hours,
(b) for a period of 7-10 days,
(c) until joint function is restored,
(d) until the inflammation is reduced and pain subsides.

2 Which one of the following remains the drug of choice for treating rheumatoid arthritis?
(a) aspirin,
(b) prednisolone,
(c) indomethacin,
(d) phenylbutazone.

1

3   Which one of the following should be used to maintain good joint position
    for Mr Franks during the night?
    (a) daily hydrotherapy,
    (b) judicious use of sandbags,
    (c) individually made splints,
    (d) well applied supportive bandages.

4   Which one of the following allows heat to be applied to Mr Franks hands?
    (a) plaster of Paris splints,
    (b) faradic baths,
    (c) hydrotherapy,
    (d) wax baths.

5   Which of the following is the most influential factor when considering
    treatment with steroids for Mr Franks?
    (a) he is depressed,
    (b) he is his own sole support,
    (c) his urinary output is normal,
    (d) his blood count is satisfactory.

6   Which one of the following is most likely to be responsible for Mr Franks'
    depression?
    (a) dysfunction and immobility,
    (b) swelling and dysfunction,
    (c) immobility and swelling,
    (d) pain and immobility.

ANSWERS TO EXAMPLE

Richard Franks

1 (d) Bed rest must be carefully
      prescribed in rheumatoid
      arthritis.

2 (a) The analgesic and anti-
      inflammatory effects of
      aspirin, together with an
      accurate knowledge of its
      possible side effects, makes it
      still the drug of choice.

3 (c) These splints maintain the
affected joints in a desirable
position without restricting
Mr Franks in other ways.

4 (d) The low boiling point of
wax, together with its heat-
retention properties, makes it
an ideal agent for the
application of local heat.

5 (b) Steroids remove symptoms
without altering the progress
of the disease, but in some
circumstances, as in those of
Mr Franks who lives alone,
these effects are desirable.

6 (d) When pain is added to any
other dysfunction, the likelihood of depression is
increased.

Mrs Arthur aged 79 years, was on her way home after collecting her pension when she tripped and fell. She was taken to the Accident and Emergency Department by ambulance. She was diagnosed as having a Colles' fracture. A plaster was applied and she was sent home later.

1 For which of the following reasons are fractures more common in the elderly? The elderly have a/an:
   (a) inability to consolidate bone,
   (b) higher incidence of falls,
   (c) less well balanced diet,
   (d) poor calcium absorption.

2 Which one of the following is the description given to the characteristic deformity produced by this fracture?
   (a) 'Dog leg',
   (b) 'Swan neck',
   (c) 'Dinner fork',
   (d) 'Spoon handle'.

3 Which one of the following should be applied immediately to immobilize Mrs Arthur's wrist?
   (a) a plaster of Paris cylinder from the base of her fingers to her elbow,
   (b) a backslab from her knuckles to the upper third of her forearm,
   (c) a plaster of Paris cylinder enclosing her wrist and forearm,
   (d) a bivalved plaster to allow inspections of her wrist.

4 In which of the following ways must Mrs Arthur's wrist be handled while the plaster is wet?
   (a) firmly, to provide support,
   (b) lightly, with the fingertips,
   (c) with one hand beneath the fracture site,
   (d) both hands must be used to support the weight.

5 Which of the following is the best way to help Mrs Arthur to remember the instructions she has been given? The nurse should:
   (a) face her and speak clearly,
   (b) give her simple written instructions,
   (c) giver her a letter for the District Nurse,
   (d) tell her several times to make sure that she understands.

6   Which of the following is the best advice to give Mrs Arthur if her fingers should swell after several days? To:
   (a) return to the Accident and Emergency Department for advice,
   (b) move her fingers and exercise her shoulder,
   (c) apply cold compresses to the fingers,
   (d) keep her arm in an elevation sling (St. John's sling).

7   Which of the following is the best activity to aid the recovery of Mrs Arthur's wrist?
   (a) ironing,
   (b) dusting,
   (c) knitting,
   (d) polishing.

Mrs Linda Hall   aged 35 years and the mother of two daughters, has been admitted to your ward for the removal of her bunions. Her feet have not been painful, but she is worried about what she sees as a foot deformity and complains that her shoes are constantly ruined.

1   Of which of the following should Mrs Hall be informed?
   (a) fallen arches may occur and might be painful,
   (b) there will be a necessity to wear flat-heeled shoes afterwards,
   (c) severe discomfort may arise as a result of interrupted circulation to the feet,
   (d) regular inspections by a chiropodist should be encouraged.

2   Which of the following is most likely to occur if Mrs Hall is given a cup of tea as soon as she comes round from her anaesthetic?
   (a) rehydration,
   (b) asphyxia,
   (c) vomiting,
   (d) nothing.

3   Which of the following observations should be recorded during the first postoperative day?
   (a) colour change, warmth and sensation of the toes,
   (b) toe colour, plaster shrinkage and ankle mobility,
   (c) popliteal pulse, plaster shrinkage and foot warmth,

(d) pedal and popliteal pulses and colour change in the foot.

4   Which one of the following positions should Mrs Hall be asked to adopt
    after the first 24 hours postoperatively?
    (a) sitting with her feet dependent,
    (b) sitting with her feet raised,
    (c) lying on alternate sides,
    (d) whatever she chooses.

5   Of which of the following should Mrs Hall be informed regarding her dis-
    charge? She must remain in hospital for:
    (a) 1 week, only if home circumstances are adequate,
    (b) 2 weeks, until sutures are removed,
    (c) 3 weeks, following a plaster change,
    (d) 4 weeks, when restricted walking is allowed.

6   For which of the following should Mrs Hall expect to have plaster casts on
    her feet?
    (a) 3-5 weeks,
    (b) 6-8 weeks,
    (c) 9-11 weeks,
    (d) 12-14 weeks.

7   Which of the following equipment should be loaned to Mrs Hall when she
    is discharged from hospital?
    (a) plaster protecting boots and walking sticks,
    (b) plaster protecting boots and crutches,
    (c) Denis Brown boots and Zimmer frame,
    (d) a plaster sock and tripod.

8   Which of the following should Mrs Hall be advised regarding the purchase
    of shoes? That:
    (a) only flat-heeled shoes must be worn,
    (b) toeless shoes are to be preferred as they are less restricting,
    (c) it might be more difficult to find comfortable shoes initially,
    (d) it is best to buy larger shoes with a laced support as they allow for
        swelling.

Colin Davis   aged 25 years, suffered a fracture dislocation of the fifth and sixth cervical spine when he dived into a swimming pool. He is quadriplegic and being nursed on a Stryker frame and with skeletal traction using skull tongs.

1   With which of the following is Colin's fracture dislocation most likely to be reduced?
   (a) spinal surgery,
   (b) cervical collar,
   (c) skeletal traction,
   (d) halo skeletal fixation.

2   Which of the following is the best reply to give Colin if he asks 'How long will I be in traction?'.
   (a) it's variable,
   (b) a minimum of 6 weeks,
   (c) about 2 weeks is usual,
   (d) I'll ask the doctor for you.

3   Which of the following is the most important observation for the nurse to make with regard to Colin's airway?
   (a) his chest expansion,
   (b) his respiratory rate,
   (c) presence of cyanosis,
   (d) the effectiveness of his cough.

4   Which of the following is the most common complication of the spinal injury Colin has received?
   (a) acute gastric dilatation and paralytic ileus,
   (b) retroperitoneal haemorrhage,
   (c) urinary tract infection,
   (d) cord compression.

5   Which of the following is the most likely cause of Colin very quickly developing pressure sores?
   (a) he cannot move himself,
   (b) spinal shock causes inadequate peripheral circulation,
   (c) the skin is denervated and thus vulnerable to pressure,
   (d) he is incontinent and skin breaks down quicker when soiled.

6   For which of the following reasons should Colin be sat up only gradually,
    once his spine is stable?
    (a) intervertebral discs are freed from stress only when the patient is hori-
        zontal,
    (b) his middle ear is not adjusted to the change and he will suffer vertigo
        and nausea,
    (c) Colin lacks vasomotor tone in his lower extremities and will become
        hypotensive in the upright position,
    (d) exaggerated autonomic responses will occur from the change in posi-
        tion leading to hypertension and hyperthermia.

7   Which one of the following should Colin be taught first, once active rehab-
    ilitation is begun?
    (a) lumbar flexion exercises to strengthen diaphragmatic movement,
    (b) muscle strengthening exercises of his feet and legs,
    (c) the psychological significance of his disability,
    (d) maintenance of sitting balance.

8   Which of the following show that Colin is developing maladaptive
    responses to his injury?
    (a) neglect and noncompliance with his therapeutic programme,
    (b) loss of self-esteem and sexual identity,
    (c) shock, denial, depression and grief,
    (d) denial of his disability.

Sara   is Mr and Mrs Rowe's first child. Just before Mrs Rowe's discharge
from the maternity unit the Paediatrician examines Sara and suspects a con-
genital dislocation of the right hip.

1   Which of the following signs will confirm the doctor's diagnosis?
    (a) adduction is limited on the right side when Sara's knees and hips are
        flexed,
    (b) the right leg appears shorter than the left,
    (c) Sara cries when the doctor abducts her hip,
    (d) there is abduction of Sara's right knee.

2   Which one of the following will be the best explanation of this condition to give the junior nurse? It occurs when:

     (a) the acetabulum fails to develop and cannot accommodate the head of the femur,

     (b) malabsorption of the head of the femur makes it too small to fit into the acetabulum,

     (c) the head of the femur slips out of the acetabulum because of a weakness of the capsule ligaments,

     (d) the upper rim of the acetabulum of the head fails to develop and there is malabsorption of the femur.

3   Which of the following is the length of time Mrs Rowe should expect Sara to remain in her Barlow's splint?

     (a) 4-8 weeks,

     (b) 8-12 weeks,

     (c) 12-16 weeks,

     (d) 16-20 weeks.

4   Which of the following is the best advice to give Mrs Rowe about caring for Sara while she is wearing her Barlow's splint?

     (a) the splint may be removed for washing purposes only,

     (b) after the initial fitting no further adjustment will be necessary,

     (c) the splint must be adjusted for the next 3 months until the leg is straight,

     (d) care must be taken to ensure that the hip should be kept at the position shown, i.e. at right angles.

5   Which of the following is the best advice to give Mrs Rowe if she finds the splint rubs Sara's skin?

     (a) adjust the splint each day so that a different area of skin is subjected to pressure,

     (b) place a good layer of cotton wool between the skin and the splint,

     (c) remove the splint and apply zinc and caster oil ointment,

     (d) leave the area exposed for an hour each day.

6   Which of the following is the best answer to give Mr and Mrs Rowe when they ask about Sara's immediate future?

     (a) no further treatment should be necessary following the application of the Barlow splint,

(b) she will need a further 6 months in plaster of Paris until the hip has grown,
(c) she will require intensive physiotherapy following splintage,
(d) she may need surgery when she is 3 years old.

7   Which of the following is the best answer to give Mrs Rowe when she asks 'Will this have any effect on her when she is grown up?'. Yes:
   (a) she may always have a slight limp on her right side,
   (b) she may develop osteoarthrosis of the right hip when she is older,
   (c) she will probably have to have corrective surgery once she has finished growing,
   (d) the hip joint will always be weak so she may not be able to carry on sporting activities.

Terry Haigh   is a 20-year-old football enthusiast and plays regularly for his local team. He was practising one evening when his knee suddenly 'locked'. His doctor, suspecting a damaged cartilage, arranged for an X-ray.

1   Which one of the following is the most likely cause of Terry's damaged cartilage? It is due to:
   (a) damage to the joint capsule,
   (b) weakening of the quadriceps muscle,
   (c) repeated tackling of other players,
   (d) twisting and turning while running.

2   Which of the following is the main aim of Terry's treatment following surgery? To:
   (a) prevent joint stiffness,
   (b) keep the leg straight to aid healing,
   (c) prevent dislocation of the other meniscus,
   (d) keep the knee straight until any effusion has subsided.

3   Which of the following is an essential part of Terry's rehabilitation following meniscectomy?
   (a) lying prone twice daily,
   (b) weight bearing after 24 hours,

10

(c) hamstring exercises three times a day,

(d) quadriceps exercises as soon as possible.

4   Which of the following is the best advice to give Terry on his discharge home?

(a) exercise regularly if your knee is not swollen,

(b) do not play football for 6 months,

(c) consider taking up another sport,

(d) always wear a support bandage.

5   Which of the following is the best answer to give Terry when he asks 'When can I start playing football again?'. When:

(a) the swelling subsides,

(b) there is no further pain,

(c) the quadriceps muscles regain their strength,

(d) you have seen the doctor 3 months after the operation.

6   Which one of the following is the best answer to give Terry when he asks 'Is my other knee likely to be affected?'.

(a) it is likely to if you continue to play football,

(b) I'm afraid you should give up playing football,

(c) it often occurs in both knees,

(d) no, it is most unlikely.

Andrew Gibson   is 12 years old and, following treatment for a compound fracture of his tibia and fibula, he is readmitted to the ward with suspected acute osteomyelitis.

1   Which of the following is the most common causitive organism?

(a) *Escherichia coli,*

(b) *Staphylococcus albus,*

(c) *Staphylococcus aureus,*

(d) *Streptococcus viridans.*

2   Which of the following is a result of osteomyelitis?

(a) sequestrum formation,

(b) absence of growth,

(c) septicaemia,

(d) fat emboli.

3   Which of the following should be the main aim of Andrew's nursing care?
    To:
    (a) provide diversional therapy,
    (b) monitor infection by taking daily swabs,
    (c) support his leg and disturb it as little as possible,
    (d) avoid stiffness of the knee by encouraging exercises.

4   Which of the following is the best advice to give Andrew's parents
    regarding his prognosis?
    (a) it takes time for the infection to resolve and he will have to rest his leg,
    (b) the pin and plates he had inserted will have to be replaced,
    (c) after the course of antibiotics his leg should be better,
    (d) the infection could re-occur elsewhere in his body.

5   Which one of the following treatments is Andrew most likely to receive if
    sequestrum forms?
    (a) local antibiotics and bone graft,
    (b) drainage and local antibiotics,
    (c) bone graft and immobilization,
    (d) immobilization and drainage.

6   Which one of the following is the reason for osteomyelitis being slow to
    respond to chemotherapy?
    (a) few antibiotics are effective against osteomyelitis,
    (b) difficulty in maintaining accurate blood levels,
    (c) neutrophils cannot penetrate compact bone,
    (d) bone has a dense cellular structure.

7   Which one of the following is the reason for Andrew's persistent pain? It is
    due to:
    (a) his reduced output of endorphins,
    (b) infiltration to the yellow bone marrow,
    (c) pressure on the nerves in the Haversian system,
    (d) the physiological response involving the periosteum.

John Barratt   aged 16 years, recently noticed a small painful swelling near
his right knee after playing football. He mentioned it to his mother when it
seemed to be enlarging and causing him considerable discomfort. His G.P.

arranged X-rays which indicate an osteogenic sarcoma. John has now to be prepared for an above-knee amputation followed by chemotherapy.

1   For which of the following reasons does John require immediate surgery?
    (a) secondary deposits in the lung rapidly occur in osteogenic sarcoma and surgery should prevent this,
    (b) spontaneous fractures will occur at the site of the tumour if amputation is delayed unnecessarily,
    (c) it is best to remove the limb before all the implications of such action are fully apparent to the patient as less distress results,
    (d) the prognosis is very good in this condition and, if treated very early, it may only require excision rather than amputation?

2   Which one of the following is likely to be of most benefit to John once he has been told he is to have amputation
    (a) discussion with a young amputee,
    (b) a visit to a limb-fitting centre,
    (c) counselling from a young people's adviser,
    (d) leave him and his parents to offer support to each other.

3   Which of the following should prevent John developing flexion contracture of the hip following amputation?
    (a) early ambulation,
    (b) lying recumbent once a day,
    (c) lying prone three times a day,
    (d) 'push-up' exercises while lying on his abdomen.

4   Which of the following is the best description of phantom limb pain to give John? It is:
    (a) an inability to tolerate a prosthesis,
    (b) persistent pain at the end of the stump,
    (c) intractable pain in the remainder of the limb,
    (d) a sensation that the limb is in its normal position.

5   Which of the following should you recommend if John asks what exercises he should carry out to strengthen his triceps?
    (a) push the thighs down onto the bed, hold for 10 seconds and then relax, and repeat that every hour while awake,

(b) use the overhead 'monkey pole' to do 'pull ups',

(c) lie on your front and do 'push ups',

(b) practise straight-leg raising.

6   Which of the following should the nurse help John to do before he attempts to walk with crutches?
(a) order a wheelchair,
(b) bandage the stump correctly,
(c) allow him to use a Zimmer frame initially,
(d) only allow him to stand at first to get the feel of normal balance.

7   Which one of the following may be responsible for John's lack of co-ordination and loss of balance once chemotherapy has commenced?
(a) feelings of weakness, due to chemotherapy, means he is less able to cope with his crutches,
(b) the toxic effects of vincristine have led to peripheral neuritis,
(c) nausea and vomiting is causing a severe electrolyte disturbance,
(d) the first signs of anaemia are developing.

8   Which of the following is the best method for estimating John's pain?
(a) careful and unobtrusive observation of the patient,
(b) use a visual analogue scale as a measure,
(c) ask him at regular intervals,
(d) a nursing care history.

Mrs Jane Slade   is a health visitor. While on her way to see one of her clients, she notices a toddler in a pushchair who seems to be somewhat deformed and has a large head. Suspecting that the child may have rickets she introduces herself to the woman in charge of the toddler.

1   Which one of the following is the correct explanation of infantile rickets? There is:
(a) defective calcification of growing bone in consequence of disturbed calcium-phosphorus metabolism,
(b) a failure of absorption of calcium from the intestine and phosphate from renal tubules associated with amino-aciduria,

14

(c) osteoporotic change,

(d) a lack of vitamin D.

2 In which of the following groups is the incidence of rickets higher than normal?

(a) low-paid workers in inner-city areas,

(b) Asian immigrants in rural areas,

(c) Asian immigrants in urban areas,

(d) refugees from the Middle East.

3 Which of the following are the clinical features that should confirm Mrs Slade's suspicions? He has:

(a) enlarged epiphyses, deformity of the chest and retarded growth,

(b) knock knees, pigeon toes and barrel-shaped chest,

(c) stick-like arms and legs, enlarged frontal bones and bulging fontanelles,

(d) a sallow appearance, appears dwarfed and has failed to gain weight.

4 Which of the following investigations should a GP arrange to confirm the health visitor's suspicions?

(a) measurement of acid phosphatase,

(b) measurement of plasma calcium,

(c) X-rays of the child's wrists,

(d) a total body scan.

5 Which of the following is the best treatment for nutritional rickets? Provision of:

(a) vitamin A,

(b) vitamin D,

(c) daily 'sunshine' therapy,

(d) weaning on to an adequate diet.

6 With which of the following should the health visitor be primarily concerned for this child?

(a) education of the mother with regard to feeding practices and general care,

(b) careful monitoring and supervision of the child's dietary intake,

(c) ensuring free milk is available to the mother,

(d) obtaining a nursery school placement.

7   Which one of the following is a common long-term complication of infantile rickets?
(a) knock knees,
(b) dental caries,
(c) an increased risk of bronchopneumonia,
(d) a decreased uptake of fat-soluble vitamins.

Mrs Agnes Storey   is a 72-year-old widow who lives alone in a third-floor council flat. A neighbour calls and finds her on the floor and suspects that she has broken her hip. She calls an ambulance to take Mrs Storey to hospital.

1   Which one of the following should make you suspect Mrs Storey has fractured the neck of her left femur?
(a) shortening and crepitus,
(b) pallor, tachycardia and pain,
(c) external rotation of the foot,
(d) adduction and plantar flexion.

2   Which of the following temporary measures is most likely to be taken if Mrs Storey is not taken for surgery straight away? Immobilize:
(a) with skin traction,
(b) with plaster of Paris,
(c) her legs with sandbags,
(d) with an inflatable splint.

3   Which one of the following measures should be taken to prevent dislocation of her prosthesis?
(a) turn her from side to back only,
(b) nurse her in the semi-recumbent position,
(c) maintain the leg in the abducted position,
(d) only sit her out in a chair on the second postoperative day.

4   Which of the following is the most likely reason for replacing Mrs Storey's head of femur?
(a) the joint ligaments are also torn,
(b) because avascular necrosis has occurred,
(c) to minimize postoperative complications,
(d) osteoarthritic changes are always present in women of this age.

5 Which one of the following is the reason for a fractured neck of femur being common in the elderly? It is due to:
(a) the building-up of osteophytes,
(b) older people being unsteady on their feet,
(c) the change in oestrogen levels in elderly women,
(d) osteoporosis causing a decalcification of the bones.

6 Which of the following is essential for Mrs Storey to be able to do before she is discharged?
(a) bath herself,
(b) cook her own meals,
(c) do her own shopping,
(d) cope with the stairs.

Mrs Grace Wicken aged 44 years, is admitted in an acute phase of rheumatoid arthritis. Her husband is a sales manager and they have three teenage daughters. Mrs Wicken's pain and stiffness has been increasing steadily and she has been finding it difficult to manage at home.

1 Which of the following characterizes rheumatoid arthritis?
(a) formation of osteophytes at joint margins,
(b) disorganization of weight-bearing joints,
(c) degeneration of articular cartilage,
(d) inflammation of synovial membranes.

2 Which one of the following is the most important consideration for Mrs Wicken on admission? To give her:
(a) a bed with extra pillows to provide her knees and ankles with extra support,
(b) a position in the ward with ease of access to bathroom and toilet,
(c) a bed with a firm base,
(d) unrestricted visiting.

3 Which one of the following should be the priority when planning Mrs Wicken's care? To:
(a) administer analgesia,
(b) assist Mrs Wicken to remain independent,

(c) relieve pain and prevent contracture deformities,

(d) maintain mobility and give limb exercises 4 hourly.

4 Which one of the following is of prime importance during an acute phase of rheumatoid arthritis? To:

(a) allow her to adopt a position of maximum comfort,

(b) maintain bed rest and apply splints to her affected limbs,

(c) keep Mrs Wicken mobile during the day and apply splints at night,

(d) provide pressure area care to prevent damage to the tissues over affected joints.

5 Which of the following may be due to side effects of the cortisone prescribed for Mrs Wicken?

(a) nausea and vomiting,

(b) oedema and restlessness,

(c) urticaria and diarrhoea,

(d) haematuria and anorexia.

6 Which of the following is the reason for prescribing local applications of heat for Mrs Wicken as her condition improves? To:

(a) reduce pain and facilitate mobility,

(b) reduce joint swelling and allow more vigorous exercise,

(c) increase reabsorption of synovial fluid by encouraging blood flow,

(d) reduce inflammation by increasing capillary dilatation thus aiding the inflammatory process.

7 Which of the following measures should best help Mrs Wicken to adjust to her increasing disability?

(a) set goals and objectives and help her achieve them,

(b) help the family to adapt to her loss of independence,

(c) help Mrs Wicken come to terms with her restricted life style,

(d) involve her fully in identifying and achieving her own goals.

Mrs Dorman   aged 50, is admitted as a 'day case' for surgery, following an appointment at the orthopaedic clinic where a carpal tunnel syndrome was diagnosed.

1   Which of the following is the best explanation to give the nurse when she
    asks 'What is carpal tunnel syndrome?'. It is due to:
    (a) flexion deformity due to contraction of the palmar fascia,
    (b) compression of the median nerve due to fibrosis,
    (c) a dislocation of the bones in her right wrist,
    (d) arthritic changes in the metacarpals.

2   Which of the following clinical features will Mrs Dorman have described
    to the doctor? That she has pain and:
    (a) tends to drop things when she uses her right hand,
    (b) she is unable to straighten her little and ring fingers,
    (c) has 'pins and needles' in her thumb, index and middle fingers,
    (d) her right hand tends to shake and she has difficulty in writing.

3   Which one of the following is the correct answer to give Mrs Dorman
    when she asks what the operation entails? It is:
    (a) splitting the palmar fascia,
    (b) division of the carpal ligaments,
    (c) division of the nerves in her right hand,
    (d) repositioning of the carpal bones in her wrist.

4   Which one of the following is the best advice to give Mrs Dorman
    following the operation?
    (a) return to out patients for removal of her stitches in 3 days time,
    (b) wear the elevation sling (St. John's sling) until the stitches are
        removed in 7 days,
    (c) wear the tubi-grip bandage until the scar has healed,
    (d) wear rubber gloves when doing the washing-up.

5   Which one of the following is the most likely cause of Mrs Dorman's con-
    dition? It is due to:
    (a) increased movement of her wrist,
    (b) osteoporosis of the carpal bones,
    (c) hormonal changes at the menopause,
    (d) synovitis of the wrist joint capsule.

6   Which of the following is the best advice to give Mrs Dorman when the
    stitches have been removed?
    (a) wear the tubi-grip bandage when she does the housework,

(b) continue to wear the sling for a further 2 weeks,
(c) avoid writing and sewing for 6 months,
(d) continue to exercise her fingers.

Gary Taylor   aged 20, is to be admitted to your ward following application of a plaster of Paris cast as treatment of his fractured tibia and fibula.

1   Of which of the following will Gary be aware after the initial application of his plaster of Paris? A sensation of:
(a) coldness due to the evaporation of the water,
(b) wetness until the plaster dries,
(c) tightness as the plaster dries,
(d) warmth when first applied.

2   Which one of the following is the best way for the nurse to handle Gary's plaster while it is still wet?
(a) gently grasping with both hands,
(b) handling with finger tips only,
(c) grip firmly at ankle and knee,
(d) using the palms of both hands.

3   Which one of the following is the best position for Gary's leg when he returns from theatre?
(a) elevate the leg on a plastic-covered pillow,
(b) support limb on either side with sandbags,
(c) leave the leg flat to maintain alignment,
(d) maintain the ankle at a right angle.

4   Which one of the following is the most appropriate action for the staff nurse to take when Gary complains of pain in his leg?
(a) elevate the leg,
(b) notify the doctor,
(c) bivalve the plaster,
(d) give analgesia as prescribed.

5   Which one of the following is the most important observation to make of Gary's foot? Evidence of:

(a) redness,
(b) sweating,
(c) numbness,
(d) irritation.

6 Which one of the following is the best answer to give Gary if he asks, 'When will I be able to walk?'.
(a) after 48 hours with the aid of crutches,
(b) after 4 weeks when the X-ray shows bone healing,
(c) after about 6 weeks when the fracture has healed,
(d) in 10 days time when they apply a 'walking' plaster.

Karen Peters is a 19-year-old student nurse who is at the end of her first year of general nurse training. During a ward placement Karen was forced to obtain 12 weeks sick leave because of a back injury.

1 Which of the following is most likely to be true of Karen's back injury? It:
(a) was avoidable,
(b) was unavoidable,
(c) is the responsibility of the ward sister,
(d) is the responsibility of the employing authority.

2 Which one of the following weights is Karen legally allowed to lift?
(a) unstipulated,
(b) 10-15 kg,
(c) 16-20 kg,
(d) 21-25 kg.

3 Which one of the following is the employing authority legally obliged to supply?
(a) a wheelchair,
(b) a 'monkey pole,'
(c) a mechanical lift,
(d) a mechanical hoist.

4 Which one of the following decisions ought Karen make regarding her future behaviour? To:
(a) avoid lifting heavy patients whenever it is possible to do so,

(b) lift heavy patients only when one or more nurses are available to assist,
(c) lift heavy patients only when the hoist is available,
(d) lift heavy patients whenever required to do so.

5   Which of the following should have prevented Karen's injury?
(a) supervision while lifting,
(b) practice sessions on lifting,
(c) insistence on using the hoist when lifting,
(d) information on the maximum weight to be lifted.

6   Which one of the following is the best way to relieve Karen's back pain?
(a) sleeping on a firm mattress,
(b) regular analgesia and physiotherapy,
(c) total absence of lifting and regular analgesia,
(d) total bed rest with planned movement and sitting.

7   Which one of the following should Karen receive?
(a) full pay while on sick leave,
(b) industrial injuries benefit,
(c) industrial compensation,
(d) disability allowance.

Melanie   is just 3 years old and the second child of Mr and Mrs Penrose.
Their GP suspects Melanie may have Still's disease (chronic inflammatory
polyarthritis) and admits her to the paediatric ward for investigations.

1   Which of the following are early features of Melanie's illness?
(a) lymphodenopathy, anaemia and a rash,
(b) rheumatoid serum factor, anaemia and a rash,
(c) early morning stiffness, anaemia and pyrexia,
(d) pyrexia, early morning stiffness and osteomalacia.

2   Which one of the following should be the main aim in caring for Melanie
during the acute stage of her illness?
(a) mobilization to prevent deformity,
(b) administration of regular analgesics,
(c) adequate rest and attention to posture,
(d) frequent tepid sponging to reduce pyrexia.

3 Which one of the following is the most likely drug therapy for Melanie?
(a) soluble aspirin,
(b) butazolidin,
(c) cortisone,
(d) Myocrisin.

4 Which one of the following is the best way for the nurse to involve Melanie's parents in her care?
(a) encourage her to mix with the other children on the ward,
(b) ask them to read to her when they visit,
(c) play with her in the bath at night,
(d) teach them to apply her splints.

5 Which one of the following is the best answer to give Mrs Penrose who asks 'How much can I let Melanie do when she comes home?' Allow her:
(a) to rest as much as possible,
(b) to ride her bicycle regularly,
(c) to play all the games that she used to,
(d) avoid games that involve her painful joints.

6 Which of the following is the most appropriate advice for the doctor to give Melanie's parents? Melanie should:
(a) continue on her drugs for the next 18 months,
(b) avoid crowded places where she is likely to pick up infections,
(c) continue with the physiotherapy sessions on a regular basis,
(d) avoid temperature extremes by keeping the house constantly warm.

7 Which one of the following is the best answer to give Melanie's parents when they ask 'How disabled will my daughter become over the next few years?'.
(a) she will become totally dependent on you for her daily care,
(b) she will be up and running around with her friends in no time,
(c) it is very probable that she will require a wheelchair by the time she is an adult,
(d) it is difficult to say because the course of the disease is variable, but being so young is an advantage.

Helen Sutton   is a 38-year-old wife and mother of 8-year-old twins. She has been admitted to your ward for terminal care having suffered from multiple myeloma for $2\frac{1}{2}$ years. All active treatment has ceased.

1   Which one of the following positions should be encouraged for Mrs Sutton now that transfusions have ceased?
(a) recumbent with one pillow if she finds this comfortable,
(b) left lateral lest she become drowsy,
(c) semi-recumbent at an angle of 45°,
(d) any position, but frequent change.

2   Which one of the following answers should you give either of her children who have asked 'Is my mummy coming home soon?'.
(a) 'I don't know,'
(b) 'Let's go and see what daddy says,'
(c) 'I'll have to ask the doctor for you,'
(d) 'we're doing our best so that she can.'

3   Which one of the following observations will still be carefully recorded for Mrs Sutton?
(a) blood pressure,
(b) urinary output,
(c) abdominal girth,
(d) level of consciousness.

4   Which one of the following diets should be provided for Mrs Sutton?
(a) liquidized food with added fibre,
(b) high protein and high calorie,
(c) low protein and high calorie,
(d) fat-free and low sodium.

5   Which one of the following programmes should be planned regarding Mrs Sutton's activity?
(a) whatever she suggests,
(b) bed rest and physiotherapy,
(c) up in a chair for the afternoon,
(d) varied according to the previous day's assessment.

24

6   Which one of the following is most likely to encourage Mrs Sutton to meet her spiritual needs?
(a) an introduction to the hospital chaplain,
(b) whatever her husband sees as helpful for her,
(c) check her history admission sheet for the correct information,
(d) a card left by her bedside so that she may make her own request to the chaplain.

Mrs Pamela Hills   is 73 years old. She fractured the head of her right femur in a fall at home. The fracture was pinned and she has made a good recovery. Mrs Hills' married daughter, Rosemary, is taking her Mother to stay with her on discharge from hospital and discusses with the Ward Sister the best arrangements to make. There is a ground-floor bedroom, bathroom and lavatory in Rosemary's home. Mrs Hills has failing eyesight but, until her accident, had been mobile and independent.

1   Which of the following is the best reply for Sister to give when Rosemary asks 'How should I arrange Mother's room for safety?' 'You should':
(a) 'remove the rugs and have polished floors only,'
(b) 'fit a handrail up the stairs in addition to the bannister,'
(c) 'leave plenty of space between the furniture for her to walk,'
(d) 'make sure that electric wires across the floor can easily be seen.'

2   Which of the following is the best reply for Sister to give Rosemary when she asks 'Will mother be able to manage using the lavatory?' 'Yes, but':
(a) 'give her a torch,'
(b) 'leave a light on in the hall,'
(c) 'leave a light on in the bedroom,'
(d) 'put her glasses where she can reach them.'

3   Which of the following is the best reply for Sister to give Rosemary when she asks 'Will Mother be able to manage using the lavatory?' 'Yes, but:'
(a) 'arrange to hire a raised toilet seat,'
(b) 'leave her a slipper bedpan at night,'
(c) 'you should borrow a commode as well,'
(d) 'fit a handle to the bathroom wall.'

4   Which of the following is the best reply for Sister to give Rosemary when
    she asks 'Can Mother have a bath?'. 'Yes, but she should be':
    (a) 'helped to stand up,'
    (b) 'allowed to sit on a stool,'
    (c) 'encouraged to take a shower instead,'
    (d) 'encouraged to use a non-slip bath mat.'

5   Which of the following is the best explanation to give Rosemary when she
    says 'Mother seems to have become "difficult" since she has been in hos-
    pital. What has happened?.' 'She':
    (a) 'is afraid of falling,'
    (b) 'doesn't like it here,'
    (c) 'is tired of doing her exercises,'
    (d) 'fears that she will never be fully mobile again.'

Colin   aged 23, was involved in a road traffic accident 7 days ago. He was
found to have a fracture of the shaft of his right femur and right radius and
ulnar. His condition suddenly deteriorated and the doctor suspects fat emboli.

1   Which one of the following best describes the term fat emboli?
    (a) hypercholesterolaemia,
    (b) fatty plaques lining the arteries,
    (c) excess lipid deposits in the veins,
    (d) the release of fat globules from the bone marrow.

2   Which one of the following would first alert the nurse to this condition?
    Colin would:
    (a) become agitated, confused and be drowsy,
    (b) have severe pain in the area of the fracture,
    (c) become hypertensive, have tachycardia and be sweating,
    (d) discolouration and loss of sensation in the affected leg.

3   Which one of the following may the nurse notice regarding Colin's
    condition?
    (a) a subnormal temperature,
    (b) peripheral cyanosis,
    (c) periods of apnoea,
    (d) a petechial rash.

4   Which one of the following actions should the nurse take while waiting for the doctor?
(a) keep Colin warm,
(b) administer oxygen,
(c) elevate the foot of the bed,
(d) give analgesic as prescribed.

5   Which one of the following is the main aim of Colin's treatment?
(a) keep him sedated until the acute stage is over,
(b) improve ventilation and reduce alkalosis,
(c) administer drugs to disperse the emboli,
(d) maintain analgesia to control pain.

6   Which one of the following is the best reply to give Colin's parents when they ask about the prognosis?
(a) once over the first 48 hours he should recover completely,
(b) he should recover, but could remain in a coma for many months,
(c) if his condition does not improve, his right leg may have to be amputated,
(d) he may require an operation to remove the fat emboli.

Mrs Jarvis   aged 69 years, has had an arthroplasty of her left hip and is now ready for discharge home. She lives with her sister in a semi-detached home in the suburbs of the city. She is apprehensive about going home and voices her fears to the Staff Nurse.

1   Which one of the following answers should the Staff Nurse give when Mrs Jarvis asks 'Is there any special way I should sleep until I come for my appointment in out-patients?.' 'It would be better if you slept':
(a) 'in a sitting position supported by three pillows,'
(b) 'on your back with your left leg supported on a pillow,'
(c) 'on your right side with a pillow supporting your left leg,'
(d) 'on your right side with a pillow in the small of your back.'

2   Which of the following is the best reply to give Mrs Jarvis when she asks 'Which kind of chair will it be most suitable for me to sit in?'. 'A chair with':
(a) 'firm arms,'

(b) 'a low seat,'
(c) 'a high back,'
(d) 'a fixed footrest.'

3   Which of the following is the best reply to give Mrs Jarvis when she asks
    'Which is the best way to get up from my chair?' 'Move to the front of your
    chair and put your':
    (a) 'left leg in front of your right,'
    (b) 'right leg in front of your left,'
    (c) 'feet apart and parallel,'
    (d) 'feet together.'

4   Which of the following is the best reply to give Mrs Jarvis when she asks
    'How should I try to walk?' 'Your steps should be':
    (a) 'long,'
    (b) 'small,'
    (c) 'straight,'
    (d) 'swinging.'

5   Which of the following is the best reply to give Mrs Jarvis when she asks
    'Can I help my sister with the housework?' 'It is best to avoid':
    (a) 'lifting furniture,'
    (b) 'standing for too long,'
    (c) 'reaching high cupboards,'
    (d) 'stooping to low cupboards.'

Adrian Jeffers   is a 33-year-old sales representative. He has consulted his
GP as he has found increasing difficulty in turning his head, particularly
when driving his car. A diagnosis of ankylosing spondylitis has been made.

1   Which of the following is the best explanation of the term 'ankylosing
    spondylitis' to give Mr Jeffers? It is:
    (a) a generalized inflammatory disease of the spinal ligaments and discs,
    (b) a weakness in the cartilaginous end plates of the vertebra allowing
        multiple protrusions of the nucleus pulposus,
    (c) slipping forward of some of the vertebra, particularly in the neck, giv-
        ing rise to pressure on nerve roots,
    (d) a generalized degenerative disc disease.

2   Which of the following are the common signs and symptoms of ankylosing spondylitis?
    (a) pain, stiffness, kyphosis and ligamentous ossification,
    (b) vertebral displacement, spinal cord damage and paraplegia,
    (c) progressive torticollis, pain and weakness of the pectoral girdle,
    (d) neck stiffness, scoliosis, osteomalacia and crepitation of the vertebral bodies.

3   Which of the following should Mr Jeffers receive initially?
    (a) lumbar osteotomy, spinal brace and physiotherapy,
    (b) spinal fusion, spinal brace and physiotherapy,
    (c) skin traction, physiotherapy and analgesia,
    (d) analgesia, physiotherapy and exercises.

4   For which of the following reasons is Mr Jeffers more prone to chest infections?
    (a) the phrenic nerves are often involved, so limiting diaphragmatic movement,
    (b) he will be confined to bed initially in a supine position,
    (c) the disease causes limitation of rib movements,
    (d) coughing is painful.

5. Which one of the following is the main approach used to manage Mr Jeffers' condition?
    (a) encouragement of sporting and other muscle-building activities,
    (b) retraining and resettlement after surgery,
    (c) prevention of extreme deformity,
    (d) early acceptance of disability.

6   Which one of the following should Mr Jeffers be recommended to carry out?
    (a) jog at least one mile a day,
    (b) lie prone for half an hour twice daily,
    (c) sleep more upright at night to limit chest infections,
    (d) register as partially disabled in order to obtain benefit.

7   Which of the following postures should Mr Jeffers be encouraged to adopt
    when sitting?
    (a) sink back into the chair to ease his lumbar spine,
    (b) bolt upright without leaning on the arms of the chair,
    (c) stretch out his legs and lean back into the chair thus supporting his
        head,
    (d) sit with a cushion in the small of his back and his elbows on the arms of
        the chair.

Jenny   aged 13, is camping with the Girl Guides. During a nature walk with
her friend she stumbles and sprains her ankle.

1   Which one of the following is the correct definition of a sprain? It is a:
    (a) dislocation of the ankle joint,
    (b) rupture of the tendons surrounding the ankle joint,
    (c) injury to the ligaments caused by wrenching or twisting,
    (d) damage to the achilles tendon by wrenching or twisting.

2   Which one of the following should be the first action that Jenny's friend
    should take?
    (a) send for medical aid,
    (b) return to the camp for help,
    (c) help Jenny back to the camp site,
    (d) sit Jenny down and elevate the foot.

3   Which one of the following is the reason for the rapid swelling of Jenny's
    ankle? It is due to:
    (a) extra vasation of blood within the tissues,
    (b) alteration in general tissue perfusion,
    (c) injury to the ankle joint capsule,
    (d) contusion of the damaged tissues.

4   Which one of the following should be the first-aid treatment for Jenny's
    ankle on return to the camp site? Apply:
    (a) cold compresses intermittently,
    (b) a crèpe bandage firmly,
    (c) a firm elastic bandage,
    (d) an elastic stocking.

5 Which one of the following will be the later treatment for Jenny's ankle?
   (a) elastic stocking and passive exercises,
   (b) complete bed rest with foot elevated,
   (c) a walking plaster will be applied,
   (d) strapping from toe to knee.

6 Which one of the following would be the best information to give Jenny
   regarding her ankle? *Full* recovery will be in approximately:
   (a) 1-2 weeks,
   (b) 3-5 weeks,
   (c) 6-11 weeks,
   (d) 12-24 weeks.

7 Which of the following is the best advice to give Jenny so that it is less likely
   to happen again?
   (a) avoid walking on uneven ground,
   (b) wear shoes which are supportive,
   (c) always wear a supportive bandage,
   (d) avoid walking very long distances.

Mr Barry Conran   a 35-year-old labourer, has been admitted with a
prolapsed intervertebral disc for assessment and possible laminectomy.
Subsequently, a myelogram revealed a prolapsed disc at level L4/L5. He has
low back pain and right-sided sciatica.

1 Which of the following is the best explanation to give a senior student
   nurse who asks 'What is a laminectomy?' It is removal of:
   (a) the lamina and the compressed nerve root,
   (b) all or part of the offending vertebral body,
   (c) the neural arch between the spinous and transverse processes,
   (d) the posterior elements of the spinal canal and the affected nerve roots.

2 Which of the following is the best explanation to give a senior student
   nurse who asks 'What is a myelogram?' It is:
   (a) an X-ray of the spinal cord,
   (b) a special X-ray of the epidural space,

(c) a radio-opaque dye injected into the subarachnoid space, the flow of which is assessed,

(d) an X-ray used to measure the amount of scoliosis present as a result of spondylitis.

3   In which one of the following positions should Mr Conran be nursed following his myelogram using Myodil?
    (a) supine,
    (b) sitting upright,
    (c) upright with bed-end raised,
    (d) supine with bed-head raised.

4   For which one of the following reasons does Mr Conran have right-sided sciatica? The prolapsed lumbar intervertebral disc is:
    (a) nipping the cauda equina,
    (b) protruding into the lamina,
    (c) pressing on a spinal nerve,
    (d) compressing a root ganglion.

5   Which one of the following exercises is likely to cause Mr Conran the most pain?
    (a) plantar flexion and extension,
    (b) hamstring contractions,
    (c) straight-leg raising,
    (d) press-ups.

6   Which of the following is the most important to ensure regarding Mr Conran's postoperative care? He:
    (a) drinks 2 litres of fluid a day,
    (b) does regular deep-breathing exercises,
    (c) performs quadriceps isometrics hourly,
    (d) keeps his shoulders and pelvis in line when turning.

7   Which of the following observations is the most important with regard to Mr Conran's recovery?
    (a) feet and legs for colour, warmth and sensation,
    (b) bladder and bowel function,
    (c) assessment of pain level,
    (d) blood pressure.

8   Which of the following is the most important arrangement that needs to be made prior to Mr Conran's return home?
    (a) he has knowledge of maximum 'loads' for his weight and height,
    (b) provision of postural supports,
    (c) he obtains a firm-based bed,
    (d) an out-patient appointment.

Mrs Gordon   aged 71 years, has suffered from osteoarthrosis of the knees for several years. She lives alone and is now only able to move around the house.

1   Which one of the following is the definition of the term osteoarthrosis? It is:
    (a) inflammation of the synovial capsule,
    (b) degeneration of the synovial capsule,
    (c) degeneration of the articulating cartilage and the development of osteophytes,
    (d) inflammation of the articulating cartilage and the development of osteatoma.
2   Which of the following is most likely to be associated with her osteo-arthrosis?
    (a) her knees feel warm to the touch when the pain is bad,
    (b) she is very stiff when she gets up in the morning,
    (c) she feels better when she's walking,
    (d) her pain is reduced after exercise.
3   Which one of the following is the best advice to give Mrs Gordon who wants to stay as active as possible?
    (a) 'rest for periods to avoid any residual stiffness',
    (b) 'increase your mobility to minimize the symptoms',
    (c) 'exercise regularly when the swelling subsides',
    (d) 'rest for long periods with your legs elevated'.
4   Which one of the following is most likely to be prescribed by Mrs Gordon's GP?
    (a) indomethacin,
    (b) prednisolone,

(c) dihydrocodeine,

(d) soluble aspirin.

5   Which one of the following is the most likely treatment when Mrs Gordon
     develops an effusion of her right knee? To:

     (a) have an arthroscopy to assess the damage,

     (b) release the fluid by intra-articular drainage,

     (c) have an intra-articular injection of steroids,

     (d) be given anti-inflammatory drugs intramuscularly.

6   Which one of the following should be the long-term aim of Mrs Gordon's
     treatment? To:

     (a) prevent deformity and minimize her pain,

     (b) encourage her to think of having a total knee replacement,

     (c) have regular physiotherapy and wear supportive knee bandages,

     (d) to arrange for help in the house and so reduce the amount she walks.

Paul Edgar   aged 30, is admitted to the accident and emergency department following a road traffic accident when his motor bike was in collision
with a taxi. He is found to have a midshaft fracture of his left femur which is to
be treated with skeletal traction.

1   Which one of the following is the correct position for the Steinman's pin in
     order to give balanced traction? It passes through the:

     (a) lower shaft of the femur,

     (b) tubercle of the tibia,

     (c) condyles of the femur,

     (d) head of the tibia.

2   Which one of the following is the reason for the foot of Paul's bed being
     raised? To:

     (a) prevent shock,

     (b) aid venous return,

     (c) provide counter traction,

     (d) prevent him slipping down the bed.

3   Which one of the following is the nurse's responsibility regarding Paul's traction?
    (a) release weights regularly to allow for physiotherapy,
    (b) reduce weights gradually as fracture heals,
    (c) keep the weights free and the ropes taut,
    (d) slacken ropes if Paul complains of pain.

4   Which one of the following is the reason for Paul's traction being discontinued?
    (a) full muscle tone has returned,
    (b) there is consolidation of bone,
    (c) he's been on a bed rest for 6 weeks,
    (d) callus formation is seen on X-ray.

5   Which one of the following is the commonest complication following a fractured shaft of femur.
    (a) fat emboli,
    (b) muscle wasting,
    (c) avascular necrosis,
    (d) deep venous thrombosis.

6   Which one of the following is the best answer to give Paul when he asks 'When can I walk without crutches?'
    (a) after 6 weeks partly bearing weight,
    (b) when the X-ray shows consolidation of bone,
    (c) after a further 6 weeks of physiotherapy,
    (d) when the thigh muscles have regained their strength.

Mr Brian Hide   aged 39 years, the managing director of a small pharmaceutical company, was feeling irritable and unwell when he arrived home at 21.00 and decided to go to bed early. He awoke at 04.00 with pain in his right big toe which rapidly worsened. By 08.00 the joint was acutely tender and Mr Hide asked his wife to send for his GP. After examining Mr Hide the GP suspects gout.

1   Which of the following is the best explanation of the term gout, to give Mr
    Hide? It is:
    (a) a degenerative change in the cartilage of the first metatarsophalangeal
        joint,
    (b) an erosive inflammatory condition of the non-weight bearing joints,
    (c) a form of septic arthritis associated with a rich diet,
    (d) an acute arthritis which results from the formation of urate crystals in
        the joint fluid.

2   Which of the following should help to confirm Mr Hide's diagnosis?
    (a) a positive rheumatoid serum factor,
    (b) a raised anti-strepsolysin (ASO) titre,
    (c) a plasma uric acid level in excess of 7 mg/100 ml^{-1},
    (d) a raised erythrocyte sedimentation rate (E.S.R.) and the presence of
        rheumatoid nodules.

3   Which of the following instructions should Mrs Hide be given regarding
    her husband?
    (a) he should stay in bed for a day and then gradually mobilize,
    (b) the affected joint must be protected from trauma — even the weight of
        the bedclothes,
    (c) 300 mg aspirin 4 hourly would control the pain and is the treatment of
        choice,
    (d) he must be forbidden to drink alcohol.

4   Which of the following is most likely to be prescribed for Mr Hide initially?
    (a) aspirin,
    (b) allopurinol,
    (c) indomethacin,
    (d) prednisolone.

5   Which of the following explanations should Mr Hide be given when he
    asks 'Will I have another attack?'
    (a) it is most unlikely if you continue to avoid alcohol,
    (b) your treatment has to be life-long and then attacks should not recur,
    (c) the development of the disease is very variable and some patients never
        have another attack,
    (d) only if you continue with your present stressful way of life and dietary
        habits.

6   Which of the following precautions should Mr Hide be asked to take if he is prescribed 'probenecid' to treat his gout? To make sure he:
(a) eats plenty of fresh fruit and vegetables,
(b) avoids cheese, red wine and marmite,
(c) maintains a good urine output,
(d) finishes the course.

7   Which of the following is a complication of untreated gout?
(a) arthritis,
(b) osteoporosis,
(c) renal failure,
(d) chondrocalcinosis.

Terry   is a 20-year-old long-distance lorry driver. He was involved in a road traffic accident which has resulted in a supracondylar fracture of his left humerus.

1   Which one of the following is most likely to be affected by this injury? The:
(a) ulnar nerve,
(b) median nerve,
(c) ulnar artery,
(d) brachial artery.

2   Which one of the following should be the initial treatment for Terry's fracture?
(a) an elevation sling (St John's sling) only,
(b) a 'gutter' plaster of Paris supported in a sling,
(c) a firm crepe pressure bandage and sling until the swelling subsides,
(d) a cylinder plaster of Paris will be applied from the wrist to the armpit.

3   Which one of the following observations must the nurse report? If:
(a) there is oedema of the forearm,
(b) the fingers appear hot, red and swollen,
(c) he complains of pain in the anticubital fossa,
(d) he complains of pain when extending his fingers.

4   Which of the following is the best reply to give Terry when he says. 'The
    doctors say I have got an ischaemic contracture?' It is:
    (a) a shortening of the muscles in your forearm,
    (b) a poor flow through the arteries of your forearm,
    (c) a shortening and thickening of the ligaments around your wrists,
    (d) the result of an impeded flow of arterial blood through your forearm.

5   Which of the following is the best answer to give Terry when he asks 'What
    is the treatment for ischaemic contracture?'
    (a) your wrist will return to normal when the fracture heals, so no further
        treatment is necessary,
    (b) you will have to go to the physiotherapy department every day and
        wear splints at night,
    (c) a collar and cuff sling will need to be worn for at least 12 weeks,
    (d) the lower arm will need to be in plaster for a further 6 weeks.

Mrs Mabel Jones   aged 78 years, has become increasingly unsteady when
walking and has fallen at home on several occasions. After lying all night on
the floor after a fall, she has been admitted to a geriatric hospital for assessment. She has osteoporosis.

1   Which of the following is the best definition of osteoporosis? It is:
    (a) a rapid bone loss due to lack of vitamin D,
    (b) a reduction in bone mass but not composition,
    (c) too little calcified bone due to inadequate vitamin D synthesis,
    (d) an imbalance between the formation and resorption of bone leading to
        a reduction in mass.

2   Which of the following statements regarding osteoporosis is correct? It is:
    (a) common in elderly men,
    (b) a feature of the ageing process,
    (c) associated with a decline in hormones,
    (d) a metabolic bone disease which is simple to treat.

3   Which of the following is directly related to Mrs Jones' diagnosis of osteo-
    porosis? She has:
    (a) lost statute and developed a kyphosis,

(b) localized back pain and some deformity,

(c) pain in her hips and pelvis and is unable to climb stairs,

(d) bone pain and tenderness, pathological fractures and difficulty in walking.

4   Which of the following is the most important aspect of the treatment of Mrs Jones' osteoporosis?

(a) analgesia for the relief of her pain,

(b) improve her mobility to delay the rate of osteoporosis,

(c) oral calcium, vitamin D and oestrogens to be prescribed,

(d) prescribed bed rest until any vertebral collapse has stabilized.

5   Which of the following groups of health care professionals should be closely involved with Mrs Jones' rehabilitation?

(a) dietician, health visitor, physiotherapist,

(b) health visitor, occupational therapist, dietician,

(c) occupational therapist, district nurse, social worker,

(d) general practitioner, physiotherapist, occupational therapist.

6   Which of the following should be recommended to Mrs Jones?

(a) a diet rich in protein, folic acid and iron,

(b) to avoid activities that could result in a fracture,

(c) to have a firm base under her mattress, i.e. a bedboard,

(d) rest is essential and braces and splints will be provided for support and reduction of muscle spasm.

Graham Morgan   is a 52-year-old batchelor who lives at home with his parents. His illness was diagnosed as multiple myeloma 18 months ago, since when he has been admitted to hospital for the correction of a pathological fracture. He is currently in your ward while he receives a course of radio-therapy.

1   Which of the following drugs are most likely to be used to reduce Graham's tumour mass and relieve his bone pain?

(a) phenylalanine mustard, cyclophosphamide and steroids,

(b) distalgesic, ferrous sulphate and nitrogen mustard,

(c) chlorambucil, pentazocine and prednisolone,

(d) vincristine, adriamycin and a salicylate.

2 Which of the following best describes multiple myelogram? It is a malignant disease that affects:
(a) lymph nodes predominantly,
(b) lymphocytes and histiocytes,
(c) the skin, by producing a pruritic red rash,
(d) plasma cells which infiltrate bone and soft tissues.

3 Which one of the following investigations should Graham undergo in order to assess the progression of his disease?
(a) liver biopsy,
(b) skeletal survey,
(c) bone marrow aspiration,
(d) blood calcium estimation.

4 Which one of the following is the most appropriate to afford Graham relief from his bone pain?
(a) cordotomy,
(b) diamorphine,
(c) acupuncture,
(d) radiotherapy.

5 To which one of the following complications is Graham particularly prone?
(a) splenomegaly,
(b) renal failure,
(c) liver intoxication,
(d) laryngeal paralysis.

6 With which of the following knowledge must Graham eventually cope? That his:
(a) prognosis is good if he takes his drugs,
(b) disease is usually fatal within 3 years,
(c) prognosis is improved if infection is controlled,
(d) life expectancy is greater now than it was 10 years ago.

Mrs Jennifer Morse   aged 39 years, has been suffering from back ache for some time and has lost a lot of time from work. Following a referral by her GP she has been admitted for a myelogram.

1   For which one of the following reasons is a myelogram performed?
    (a) compression of the spinal cord and/or spinal nerves may be detected,
    (b) the extent of demyelinating diseases can be estimated,
    (c) it measures isometric contractions in back muscles,
    (d) a diagnosis of myeloma can be confirmed.

2   Which of the following is the best reply to give Mrs Morse if she asks 'How
    long will the myelogram take?'.
    (a) 'as you'll be anaesthetized, you won't notice time passing,'
    (b) 'it depends, it will vary for each patient,'
    (c) 'oh, not long — about half an hour,'
    (d) 'normally about 1 to 2 hours.'

3   Which of the following is the best answer to give a junior student nurse
    who asks 'How is a myelogram performed?'
    (a) the patient is connected to a special machine measuring the electrical
        activity of muscles,
    (b) an epidural tap is performed and air introduced to act as a contrast to
        show on X-rays,
    (c) a lumbar puncture is performed, and a contrast medium introduced
        and its flow monitored,
    (d) a bone marrow puncture is required with X-rays of the procedure.

4   For which one of the following reasons should Mrs Morse be fasted for 4
    hours prior to the investigation.
    (a) a general anaesthetic will be given,
    (b) giddiness and nausea commonly occur,
    (c) she is less likely to develop a headache,
    (d) no blood is being diverted to the gastrointestinal system interfering
        with the results.

5   Which one of the following should Mrs Morse be warned to expect during
    the myelogram?
    (a) a pounding sensation in her head just while air is injected,
    (b) that the X-ray table will be tilted during the procedure like 'a slow-
        motion fairground ride',
    (c) she will need to remain absolutely still to avoid giving false readings,
    (d) that she will be anaesthetized while lying on the X-ray table.

6   Which of the following observations are the most important following Mrs
    Morse's myelogram?
    (a) sensation, warmth and mobility of lower limbs,
    (b) evidence of internal haemorrhage,
    (c) fluid intake and output,
    (d) complaints of headache.

7   For which of the following is a myelogram specifically contraindicated?

    (a) a married woman on 'the pill',
    (b) a teenage girl with epilepsy,
    (c) a man with Menière's disease,
    (d) a man with kyphosis.

8   Which one of the following should Mrs Morse be asked to carry out in
    order to reduce the headache she has developed 12 hours later?
    (a) drink plenty of water or squash,
    (b) adopt an upright position even while asleep,
    (c) to remain lying in a 'head down' position for 24 hours,
    (d) to get up and about as soon as all her observations are stable.

James Parry   is a 25-year-old man who has been admitted to hospital
following a road traffic accident. He is shocked but not unconscious, although
he has made no attempt to move.

1   Which one of the following is appropriate when preparing Mr Parry for
    examination by the doctor in the Accident and Emergency Department?
    (a) remove all clothes and cover with a blanket,
    (b) remove those clothes where injury is apparent,
    (c) cover with a blanket without removing any clothes,
    (d) cover with a blanket after washing the injured areas.

2   Which of the following is the most important information to obtain?
    (a) knowledge of when urine was passed,
    (b) identification to inform relatives,
    (c) identification for consent to surgery,
    (d) knowledge of when last meal was eaten.

3 Which one of the following indicates that Mr Parry may have developed
   paraplegia? An inability to move:
   (a) both arms,
   (b) both legs,
   (c) both arms and legs,
   (d) one side of his body.

4 To which one of the following hazards should the nurse be alerted when it
   is confirmed that Mr Parry is paraplegic?
   (a) frustration due to inability to hold anything firmly,
   (b) falls, due to difficulty in co-ordinating his gait,
   (c) pressure sores due to insensitivity to pain,
   (d) indigestion due to inability to chew.

5 Which of the following is most likely to enable Mr Parry to maintain his
   self-esteem?
   (a) be prepared to listen,
   (b) anticipate all his needs,
   (c) ensure he does as much as he can,
   (d) provide him with the aids available.

6 Which one of the following answers should you give Mr Parry when he
   asks, 'Will I ever be able to walk again?'
   (a) 'I'll fetch sister,'
   (b) 'I really don't know,'
   (c) 'I don't think you will,'
   (d) 'What did the doctor tell you?'

Miss Anne Briggs aged 35 years, a deputy headmistress, had been
experiencing some increasing pain and stiffness in her right knee. All other
tests having been inconclusive, she was admitted to hospital for an
arthroscopy the next morning.

1 Which of the following is the best explanation of the term arthroscopy? It
   is a/an:
   (a) experimental technique used to examine knees, hips and shoulders,
   (b) endoscopic investigation of the internal structures of a joint,

(c) thermographic technique used to detect inflammatory changes in large joints,

(d) X-ray of a joint which involves double-contrast techniques and several injections of gas into the joint space.

2 Which of the following preparations must Miss Briggs undergo prior to arthroscopy?
(a) physiotherapy for hamstring exercises,
(b) shaving of the leg and pubic area,
(c) preparation for spinal block,
(d) previous arthrogram.

3 Which of the following is the correct answer to give Miss Briggs if she asks 'How long will the arthroscopy take?'
(a) 'Only about 10 minutes,'
(b) 'It is difficult to say,'
(c) 'A minimum of 30 minutes,'
(d) 'It is only a minor operation.'

4 Which of the following is the major reason why some form of anaesthesia is normally used during the procedure? Because:
(a) a tourniquet is applied at the thigh to reduce blood flow to the knee,
(b) a fibreoptic light source has to be introduced into the joint space,
(c) the knee joint has to be distended with 100-200 ml of saline,
(d) a small incision is made in the infrapatellar region.

5 Which of the following is the most important item to include in Miss Briggs' immediate postoperative care?
(a) quadriceps exercises,
(b) observation of the dressing,
(c) checking of toes for circulation and sensation,
(d) control of postoperative pain with controlled drugs.

6 Which of the following is the most appropriate answer to give Miss Briggs if she asks 'How long do I have to stay in bed?' 'Until':
(a) 'you feel better,'
(b) 'you are fully recovered from the anaesthetic,'
(c) 'you are free of pain and can walk with crutches,'
(d) '48 hours after the investigation when there is less chance of your knee swelling.'

44

7 Which of the following instructions should Miss Briggs be given before her discharge home? To:
  (a) continue using crutches until seen in out-patients in 2 weeks time,
  (b) expect the district nurse to come to remove the stitch in 10 days,
  (c) attend physiotherapy department weekly for quadriceps exercises,
  (d) walk at least 2 miles every day.

8 Which of the following replies is the best to give Miss Briggs if she asks 'Can anything go wrong with my knee after this investigation?'
  (a) 'Your knee will be sore for a few weeks,'
  (b) 'It is unlikely, complications are very rare,'
  (c) 'Not unless you put too much weight on it too soon,'
  (d) 'You must expect your knee to be swollen and painful for a week or two.'

Mrs Barton is a 53-year-old woman who had a mastectomy operation 4 years ago and who has since developed bony metastatic deposits. She has been admitted to your ward following a fracture of her radius and ulna which is the result of an accident at home. Her frail condition is causing her husband a great deal of concern.

1 Which of the following should best help Mr Barton cope with his wife's admission? A/an:
  (a) home help,
  (b) appointment with the medical social worker,
  (c) opportunity to visit whenever he is able to do so,
  (d) suggestion that he shares the physical care of his wife.

2 Which one of the following should be elicited from Mrs Barton regarding her pain?
  (a) 'Point to where your arm hurts, please,'
  (b) 'Can you show me where the pain is?',
  (c) 'Does your arm hurt very much?,'
  (d) 'Do you have any pain?'

3 Which one of the following is essential in the healing of Mrs Barton's fracture?
  (a) calcitonin,

(b) parathormone,
(c) zinc phosphate,
(d) calcium phosphate.

4 Which of the following is most commonly the first indication of a secondary bony metastatic deposit?
(a) pain and tenderness,
(b) spontaneous fracture,
(c) lethargy due to anaemia,
(d) susceptibility to infection.

5 Which one of the following is the best answer to give when Mr Barton asks, 'How long does it usually take for this type of fracture to heal?'.
(a) 'It is unlikely that your wife's fracture will ever heal,'
(b) '10-12 weeks, but your wife's illness will probably alter that,'
(c) 'I wouldn't really like to say as far as your wife is concerned,'
(d) 'Healthy people usually have their plaster removed after 6 weeks.'

6 Which one of the following should be offered to Mrs Barton in order to reduce the possibility of her developing a urinary tract infection?
(a) complete privacy in relation to using a bed pan,
(b) vulval toilet following the use of a bed pan,
(c) correct positioning during defaecation,
(d) the use of a commode.

7 Which one of the following is the most appropriate answer to give Mr Barton when he asks your advice on whether to spend the night at the hospital, as his wife's condition has deteriorated?
(a) 'I believe it would be best if you wish to ensure being with your wife when she dies,'
(b) 'You must look after yourself properly, too, and you certainly need a night's sleep,'
(c) 'Could you come with me so that we can talk about it together?'
(d) 'Why don't you ask your wife what she would like you to do?'

ANSWERS

Mrs Arthur

1 (b) Evidence demonstrates that the aged suffer falls most frequently.

2 (c) The only correct answer.

3 (b) A backslab is sufficient to immobilize the fracture, but allows for swelling formation without the danger of circulatory restriction.

4 (d) This handling provides evenly spread pressure and avoids depressing the plaster, which could result in the indentation rubbing against the skin and causing a plaster sore.

5 (b) No assumptions should be made about Mrs Arthur's ability to remember any instruction as this is a distressing time for her and her anxiety will limit her attention.

6 (a) Swelling resulting from the injury should be subsiding at this stage, so this undue swelling reflects an inappropriately tight plaster which should only be adjusted in the

Accident and Emergency Department.

7 (c) This activity gives the greatest range of movement.

Mrs Linda Hall

1 (c) Without this information Mrs Hall may believe that such discomfort is peculiar to her and a sign that something is going wrong.

2 (c) An inevitable after effect of anaesthesia.

3 (a) These observations are essential in order to assess the circulation (or its impediment) to the foot.

4 (b) Mrs Hall's feet need to be raised in order to reduce swelling.

5 (a) One week should ensure recovery from the trauma of the surgery and the anaesthetic, and home is the best place for further recovery, providing support is available.

6 (c) 9-11 weeks is an average bone healing time for an otherwise healthy adult.

7 (b) Mrs Hall will be walking with

the aid of crutches because she will only be partially weight bearing.

8 (d) Circulatory difficulties will continue for some time.

Colin Davis

1 (c) Only traction can reduce a fracture dislocation.

2 (b) Information reduces patients' anxiety and a minimum period has been given.

3 (d) An ineffectual cough may indicate an inadequate diaphragmatic movement (spinal nerves C3, 4 and 5 innervate the diaphragm).

4 (a) Injury to the spinal cord at this level may result in decreased innervation of the stomach and small bowel.

5 (b) The low blood pressure associated with spinal shock is inadequate to maintain the desired tissue perfusion.

6 (c) A lack of vasomotor tone results in pooling of venous blood and normal blood pressure maintenance requires an adequate venous return.

7 (d) This stance is essential to Colin's understanding of the limitations imposed by his paralysis.

8 (a) This is the only maladaptive response (see Kubler Ross's work on loss).

Sara

1 (a) As the femoral head slips out of the acetabulum.

2 (c) Only correct answer.

3 (b) The usual period of time.

4 (d) This position will ensure correction without further deformity.

5 (b) Where the cause of the pressure cannot be removed its action can be ameliorated by this layer of cotton wool.

6 (a) Only correct answer.

7 (b) Any mal-positioning at joint level may predispose to osteo-arthrosis, i.e. degenerative disease.

Terry Haigh

1 (d) The most common cause in footballers.

2 (d) This position reduces pressure on the suture line.

3 (d) Firm quadriceps are essential to joint stability.

4 (a) Swelling is an indication of active inflammation which will be aggravated by exercise.

5 (c) See 3(d).

6 (a) See 1(d).

Andrew Gibson

1 (c) Only correct answer.

2 (a) Sequestrum forms as part of the inflammatory process, being composed of dead bone, fibrous tissue, etc.

3 (c) Maintenance of the correct positioning of Andrew's leg encourages healing without deformity and reduces discomfort.

4 (a) This honest answer respects both the intelligence of Andrew's parents and acknowledges their need to know.

5 (b) Sequestrum cannot be absorbed, hence drainage and antibiotics are essential to control the infection both systemically and locally.

6 (d) Systemically operative drugs can only work if the blood supply to the target area is good enough to allow for drug serum levels to be maintained as high as is required.

7 (d) Periosteum has an abundant nerve supply and thus when inflamed causes great pain.

John Barratt

1 (a) Secondary deposits are the most dangerous threat to a favourable prognosis for John and thus attempts at their prevention are therefore justified.

2 (a) The help offered by someone who understands the problem from inside is incomparable and affords John a realistic insight into the potential

problems.

3 (c) This method is currently practised at specialist limb-fitting centres.

4 (d) Only correct answer.

5 (c) Having located the triceps all students are able to test the truth of this statement.

6 (d) This will reduce the incidence of falls and their demoralizing effect, which hinders recovery.

7 (b) Only correct answer.

8 (b) A visual analogue scale, e.g. pain 'thermometer', reduces the interference of the nurse's perception in estimating John's pain.

Mrs Jane Slade

1 (a) The only totally correct answer, it is possible to have a normal vitamin intake and yet develop rickets.

2 (c) Current evidence supports this answer. It is possible that the pigmented skin of immigrants is less efficient in the synthesis of vitamin D (Dent 1969. In *Oxford Textbook of Medicine Vols 1 & 2* (1983) edited by D J Wetherall et al., Oxford University Press).

3 (a) Rachitic children show widening of the epiphyses of the long bones at growing points and the ribs become

drawn in under the pull of the diaphragm. (Hence these features).

4 (c) Such X-rays will show the characteristic rachitic changes with enlargement and irregularity of the epiphyseal plate.

5 (b) Nutritional rickets is caused by lack of vitamin D, thus vitamin D or an adequate diet is prescribed.

6 (a) Many Asian immigrants retain their customary dietary habits, which avoid vitamin D-rich foods, and thus children may become vitamin D deficient.

7 (c) Due to the chest deformity.

Mrs Agnes Storey

1 (c) Shortening adduction and external rotation of the affected leg are classic features.

2 (a) Relieves pain, immobilizes the fracture yet allows the patient some freedom of movement while in bed.

3 (c) In this position the femoral head is 'seated' firmly in the acetabulum until soft tissues have healed.

4 (b) Fractured neck of femur may disrupt the blood supply to the head of the femur leading to anoxia and necrosis (avascular).

5 (d) Only correct answer.

6 (d) She lives in a third-floor council flat and thus must be able to climb stairs even if rehousing is eventually successful.

Mrs Wicken

1 (d) Only correct answer.

2 (c) Rest while maintaining good posture to minimize joint deformity is an aim of treatment.

3 (c) Treatment is designed to modify the course of the disease and reduce the likelihood of joint deformity and consequent disability.

4 (b) See answers 2 and 3 above.

5 (b) The effects of 'salt and water' retention.

6 (a) Local applications of heat improve circulation and reduce swelling.

7 (d) Provides her with motivation to overcome disability.

Mrs Dorman

1 (b) Only correct answer.

2 (c) Due to compression of the nerve (median) which supplies these digits giving abnormal sensation.

3 (b) Correct — one hopes further explanation will follow!

4 (b) This keeps the hand elevated and encourages venous

return thus limiting swelling.
5 (c) Currently thought to be the commonest cause.
6 (d) Speeds return of full function.

Gary Taylor
1 (d) When water is added to plaster of Paris, the reaction that occurs also produces heat.
2 (d) Evenly distributes the weight and is less likely to cause indentations in the plaster.
3 (a) Reduces swelling and aids venous return.
4 (a) Reduction of swelling is likely to reduce the pain and is the *first* action to be taken.
5 (c) Implies interference with the circulation of blood and tissue anoxia.
6 (a) Only correct answer.

Karen Peters
1 (a) See recent survey on back pain *(Hazards in the Health Service — An A-Z guide* (1984) GMBATU).
2 (a) Only correct answer at the moment (see 1 (a)).
3 (d) Employing authorities who do not supply mechanical lifting aids are legally liable should back injury occur.
4 (c) This is part of what makes back injury avoidable.

5 (c) The only correct answer as the hoist is taking the strain!
6 (d) Rest is essential to healing and unregulated movements may cause pain and further damage.
7 (b) A legal right.

Melanie
1 (a) These are common systemic manifestations of Still's disease.
2 (c) Prevention of flexion deformities and a programme to maintain a full range of joint movements is essential.
3 (a) Aspirin is the most likely drug therapy — the others are only used in severe cases or if complications occur.
4 (d) Night rest splints prevent flexion deformities and are a very important part of Melanie's treatment.
5 (d) Enough activity to maintain joint movement but avoid further pain.
6 (c) A regular supervised exercise programme will help maintain a full range of joint movements.
7 (d) The prognosis is considerably better than that of the adult disease, except in a small group of patients with an erosive sero-positive polyarthritis.

51

Helen Sutton

1 (c) She will find breathing less distressing and be able to see activities in the ward.

2 (b) This does not raise false hopes and involves the father so that any answer concurs with his wishes.

3 (b) To avoid over or under-hydration and thus exacer-bating her distress.

4 (a) Easy to digest but provides roughage and reduces the likelihood of constipation.

5 (d) Nursing care should be planned according to the assessed needs of the patient.

6 (a) Allows her to receive as much or as little help as she requires with the minimum of effort.

Pamela Hills

1 (c) Only commonsense answer that is correct.

2 (b) Insufficient light to disturb her, but enough for her to distinguish outlines of objects.

3 (c) Less distance to walk during the night and thus less risk of accidents.

4 (b) Use of a bath stool aids independence.

5 (a) Has lost confidence in her own ability to manage and thus may seem 'difficult'.

Colin

1 (d) The best description.

2 (a) These are signs of the resulting hypoxia.

3 (d) A petechial rash is caused by extravasation of blood from fragile capillaries due to the presence of fat globules.

4 (b) Fat emboli will occur in lung tissue interfering with gaseous exchange, leading to tissue hypoxia.

5 (b) The alkalosis resulting from poor ventilation is life threatening.

6 (b) This is a truthful response which shows respect for Colin's parents.

Mrs Jarvis

1 (c) This position should be comfortable but at the same time maintain a good joint position and reduce the danger of dislocation.

2 (a) A chair with firm arms takes the strain when Mrs Jarvis stands, which reduces strain on the hip joint.

3 (a) This position ensures that maximum weight be taken initially on the nonoperated leg.

4 (c) Straight steps will keep the

joint in correct alignment.

5 (d) This action causes external rotation and adduction and may precipitate dislocation.

Adrian Jeffers

1 (a) Only correct answer.

2 (a) Only correct answer.

3 (d) The whole emphasis of treatment is on active mobilization and analgesia will relieve pain and allow the patient to be active.

4 (c) Respiratory movements become restricted due to involvement of the costovertebral joints limiting chest expansion.

5 (c) Immobility leads to ankylosis; activity and good posture limit deformity.

6 (b) The hip joint is commonly involved and this reduces the risk of flexion deformities.

7 (b) Maintenance of good natural position reduces the risk of deformities.

Jenny

1 (c) Only correct definition.

2 (d) Helps to limit the swelling and thus reduce pain.

3 (a) Bleeding occurs from damaged ligamentous structures surrounding the joint causing swelling.

4 (a) Vasoconstricting effects of cold retard extravasation of blood and reduce pain.

5 (d) To reduce swelling and oedema and support the damaged joint structures.

6 (d) Torn fibres and ligaments are slow to heal.

7 (b) Thus she is less likely to 'turn her ankle'.

Mr Barry Conran

1 (c) Only correct answer.

2 (c) Only correct answer.

3 (d) The contrast medium remains in the lower part of the spinal theca and spinal cord and this reduces the risk of headache.

4 (c) The nerve root involved in this instance is the sciatic nerve.

5 (c) This exercise most stretches the sciatic nerve and therefore causes extreme pain.

6 (d) This lineation will maintain reduced mobility of the spinal column and thus minimize pain and trauma.

7 (b) Innervation to the bowel and bladder is via the spinal nerves (sacral plexus) thus changes in their function might be ascribed to the healing or otherwise of a cord lesion.

8 (c) A firm-based bed reduces the

likelihood of further
postural deformities.

Mrs Gordon
1 (c) Only correct answer.
2 (c) This is a feature of
osteoarthrosis.
3 (b) This disease causes pain on
resting and thus tends to
discourage exercise, but
mobility is desirable not only
because it increases independence but because it reduces
the pain experienced.
4 (a) A nonsteroidal anti-
inflammatory drug,
particularly effective in
osteoarthrosis.
5 (c) The anti-inflammatory
effects of steroids will halt
the fluid (effusion)
formation.
6 (a) This maintains her
independence and is the least
intrusive.

Paul Edgar
1 (b) A Steinman's pin inserted
into an unstable fragment
cannot give balanced
traction. The pull is always
through a joint.
2 (c) Only correct answer.
3 (c) Only this answer falls within
the remit of the nurse.
4 (d) Callus formation is the

indication of bone healing.
5 (a) Only correct answer.
6 (b) Refracture is likely if
consolidation has not taken
place.

Mr Brian Hide
1 (d) Only correct answer.
2 (c) Over-production or insufficient excretion of urates may
cause hyperuricaemia and
subsequent gout.
3 (b) The joint becomes acutely
painful and very tender and
should be protected to
minimize the pain.
4 (c) A nonsteroidal anti-
inflammatory drug and the
least likely to exacerbate or
prolong the attack.
5 (b) Long-term drug therapy is
aimed at reducing the
production of uric acid.
6 (c) Inadequate fluid intake will
give rise to the formation of
gravel and possible renal
stones.
7 (c) Urates are desposited in
renal tubules leading to
nephropathy and renal
failure.

Terry
1 (d) See an anatomy text.
2 (b) Allows for swelling.
3 (d) This indicates pressure on

the median nerve.
4 (d) This is the fullest answer and thus a better explanation.
5 (b) Exercise and maintenance of a good position through splinting will aid recovery.

Mabel Jones
1 (d) The correct definition.
2 (b) The most common cause is ageing.
3 (a) The spine is especially affected leading to loss of height and an abnormal spinal curvature (kyphosis).
4 (b) It is thought that long-term immobilization causes osteoporosis (G A Rose 1967. In *Oxford Textbook of Medicine Vols 1 & 2* (1983) edited by D J Wetherall et al., Oxford University Press). Thus improving mobility delays the rate of progression.
5 (c) In order to keep her as independent as possible.
6 (c) Backache is a common feature and also the spine is especially prone to fractures.

Graham Morgan
1 (a) The cytotoxics named are shown to have increased survival rates (J R Hobbs 1969. In *Oxford Textbook of*

Medicine Vols 1 & 2 (1983) edited by D J Wetherall et al., Oxford University Press). Prednisolone lowers the serum calcium level and is of value in the presence of anaemia.
2 (d) The best description.
3 (c) Will show infiltration of the bone marrow with abnormal plasma cells.
4 (d) Radiotherapy relieves bone pain faster than chemotherapy, but is purely palliative.
5 (b) Due to presence of abnormal immunoglobulins which have to be excreted but clog the renal tubules.
6 (b) Prognosis is variable but still poor.

Mrs Jennifer Morse
1 (a) By outlining the spinal theca it is possible to estimate the position and extent of any lesion compressing the cord or spinal nerves.
2 (d) Need to give information to reduce anxiety.
3 (c) The correct answer.
4 (b) The correct explanation.
5 (b) Unless prewarned this could be very alarming.
6 (a) Early indicators of spinal trauma.

7 (b) A history of epilepsy is
considered to be a contra-
indication as fits will be
precipitated.

8 (a) Removal of some cerebrospinal fluid leads to traction
on cerebral blood vessels and
a headache. A good fluid
intake hastens the recovery
of normal pressure in the
cerebrospinal fluid.

James Parry

1 (c) A spinal cord injury should be
suspected and the patient
treated accordingly, i.e. the
patient should not be moved
until the suspicion is proved
groundless.

2 (b) This is the most important as
surgery is not contemplated.

3 (b) Total sensory and/or motor
loss below the level of the
injury. A paraplegia gives
paralysis of both lower limbs.

4 (c) Due to sensory loss below the
level of the spinal injury.

5 (c) Helps to satisfy his need to be
independent.

6 (d) An open question that allows
assessment of Mr Parry's
knowledge.

Miss Anne Briggs

1 (b) Only correct explanation.

2 (b) To reduce bacterial load of
skin and minimize risk of

infection.

3 (c) Adequate explanation
reduces anxiety, in this case a
minimum time has been given
in order to accom-
modate variability.

4 (c) Stretching a joint capsule is
painful.

5 (c) To ensure there is no surgical
trauma blood or nerve
supply and that post-surgical
oedema does not interfere
either.

6 (b) Patients are encouraged to
rest and then can be
mobilized with a walking
stick in the evening.

7 (b) The only further treatment
necessary until the surgeon
has decided on future treatment in the light of current
findings.

8 (b) Complications are *very* rare,
occasionally infection may
occur.

Mrs Barton

1 (c) Separation increases the possibility of alienation and this
must be guarded against
when both Mr and Mrs
Barton are experiencing,
arguably, their greatest need
for human contact.

2 (d) This answer suggests that the
nurse is making no assump-

tions about Mrs Barton's pain.

3 (a) Calcitonin is essential to calcium uptake which in turn is essential to the healing of bone.

4 (b) Only correct answer.

5 (b) This answer demonstrates the knowledge required for healing or bones in general, and also shows a desire to be honest with Mr Barton.

6 (d) The use of a commode allows for a more normal position to be maintained while voiding urine, which facilitates total emptying of the bladder and the reduction in the poss- ibility of infection arising from stagnant urine.

7 (c) This answer suggests that the nurse acknowledges that a problem exists but chooses to use this occasion to assess the need Mr Barton has of her or of anyone else's support.